STAYING HEALTHY AND AVOID CANCER:

Making a healthy living a priority

Elizabeth B Caron

Table of contents

Chapter1:

Staying healthy

A variety of factors play a part in keeping healthy. In turn, excellent health may minimize your chance of acquiring certain illnesses. These include heart disease, stroke, certain malignancies, and traumas. Learn what you can do to maintain your and your family's health.

The Path to Enhanced Health

Eat healthily.

What you consume is intimately connected to your health. Balanced nutrition offers several advantages. By adopting healthy eating choices, you may avoid or cure various diseases. These include heart disease, stroke, and diabetes. A nutritious diet may help you lose weight and lower your cholesterol as well.

Get frequent exercise.

Exercise may help avoid heart disease, strokes, diabetes, and colon cancer. It may help treat depression, osteoporosis, and high blood pressure. People who exercise also get hurt less frequently. Routine exercise may help you feel better and keep your weight under control. Try to be active for 30 to 60 minutes around 5 times a week. Remember, any quantity of activity is better than none.

If you're overweight, lose weight.
Many Americans are overweight. Carrying too much weight raises your risk for various health issues. These include:

High blood pressure, high cholesterol
Diabetes type 2
Heart disease, stroke, and certain cancers
Gallbladder disease

Being overweight might also contribute to weight-related ailments. A typical concern is arthritis in the weight-bearing joints, such as your spine, hips, or knees. There are various things you may try to help you lose weight and keep it off.

Protect your skin.

Sun exposure is connected to skin cancer. This is the most common kind of cancer in the United States. It's better to restrict your time spent in the sun. Be careful to wear protective gear and helmets while you are outdoors.

Use sunscreen year-round on exposed skin, such as your face and hands. It protects your skin and helps prevent skin cancer. Choose a broad-spectrum sunscreen that filters both UVA and UVB rays. It should be at least an SPF of 15. Do not sunbathe or use tanning booths.

Things to consider

In addition to the things outlined above, you should create time for total body wellness. Visit your physician for frequent checks. This includes your regular doctor, as well as your dentist and eye doctor.

Let your health benefits and preventative care services work for you. Make sure you know what your health insurance plan entails. Preventive treatment may identify diseases or prevent sickness before they start. This includes specific medical appointments and screenings. You need to make time for breast health.

Breast cancer is a primary cause of mortality for women. Men may acquire breast cancer, too. Talk to your doctor about when you should start receiving mammograms. You may need to start screening early if you have risk factors, such as family history. One technique to identify breast cancer is to undertake a monthly self-exam.

Women should have regular Pap smears as well. Women aged 20 to 60 should be tested every 3 years. This may change if you have specific problems or have had your cervix removed.

Ask your doctor about different cancer screenings. Adults should be checked for colorectal cancer starting at age 45 to 50. Your doctor may want to check for other forms of cancer. This will depend on your risk factors and family history.

Keep a list of the current drugs you take. You also should remain up to date on immunizations, including obtaining an annual flu vaccine. Adults require a TD booster every 10 years. Your doctor may replace it with Tdap.

This also protects against whooping cough (pertussis) (pertussis). Women who are pregnant require the TDAP immunization. People who are in close touch with newborns should receive it as well.

Chapter2:

Staying healthy

How many calories should I consume and how frequently should I exercise to maintain my present weight?
Should I get an annual physical exam?
What sorts of preventative care does my insurance cover?
When should I start being checked for various tumors and conditions?
Which healthy option is the most crucial for me?

The start of a new decade brings with it new goals to enhance one's life, including a healthier lifestyle. Here are 19 practical health recommendations to help you start out towards healthy living in 2022.

1.Eat a healthy diet

Eat a mix of various foods, including fruit, vegetables, legumes, nuts, and healthy grains. Adults should consume at least five pieces (400g) of fruit and vegetables every day. You can increase your intake of fruits and vegetables by including them in all of your meals, eating fresh fruit and vegetables as snacks, eating a variety of fruits and vegetables, and eating them in season.By eating properly, you will minimize your risk of malnutrition and noncommunicable diseases

(NCDs) such as diabetes, heart disease, stroke, and cancer.

2. Reduce your intake of salt and sugar.

Filipinos drink double the recommended amount of salt, putting them at risk of high blood pressure, which in turn raises the risk of heart disease and stroke. Most individuals receive their sodium from salt. Reduce your salt consumption to 5g per day, which is equal to around one teaspoon.

It's easy to achieve this by minimizing the quantity of salt, soy sauce, fish sauce, and other high-sodium condiments while cooking meals; eliminating salt, spices, and condiments from your dinner table;

avoiding salty snacks; and selecting low-sodium items.

On the other hand, ingesting excessive quantities of sweets raises the risk of tooth damage and unhealthy weight gain. Free sugar consumption should be limited to less than 10% of total energy intake in both adults and children.

This is comparable to 50g, or around 12 tablespoons for an adult. For added health benefits, WHO recommends consuming less than 5% of total energy consumption.You may lower your sugar intake by minimizing the use of sugary snacks, sweets, and sugar-sweetened drinks.

3. Reduce your intake of unhealthy fats.

Fat consumption should not exceed 30% of total energy intake.This will assist in avoiding unhealthy weight gain and NCDs. There are numerous kinds of fats. However, unsaturated fats are preferred over saturated fats and trans-fats. WHO recommends limiting saturated fats to less than 10% of total energy intake, limiting trans fats to less than 1% of total energy intake, and replacing both saturated and trans fats with unsaturated fats.

Saturated fats are found in fatty meat, butter, palm, and coconut oil, cream, cheese, ghee, and lard; and trans fats are found in baked and fried foods, as well as pre-packaged snacks and foods such as frozen pizza, cookies, biscuits, and cooking oils and spreads.

4.Avoid excessive alcohol consumption

There is no safe amount of alcohol to consume. Consuming alcohol may lead to health issues such as mental and behavioral disorders, including alcohol dependency; significant NCDs such as liver cirrhosis; certain cancers and heart illnesses; as well as injuries arising from violence and traffic confrontations and crashes.

5.Don't smoke

Smoking tobacco promotes NCDs such as lung disease, heart disease, and stroke. Tobacco kills not just direct smokers but also non-smokers via second-hand exposure. Currently, there are roughly 15.9 million Filipino people who smoke tobacco, although 7 in 10 smokers are interested or aim to stop.

If you are currently a smoker, it's not too late to stop. Once you do, you will enjoy instant and long-term health advantages. If you are not a smoker, that's excellent! Do not start smoking and fight for your right to breathe tobacco-smoke-free air.

6.Being active

Physical activity is defined as any physical movement generated by skeletal muscles that involves energy expenditure. This includes exercise and activities conducted while working, playing, carrying out home tasks, travelling, and indulging in leisure interests. The quantity of physical activity you require varies with your age group, but individuals aged 18–64 years should complete at least 150 minutes of moderate-intensity physical exercise throughout the week. Increase moderate-intensity physical exercise to 300 minutes per week for extra health advantages.

7.Check your blood pressure frequently.

Hypertension, or excessive blood pressure, is dubbed a "silent killer". This is because many individuals who have hypertension may not be aware of the condition since it may not have any symptoms. If left unchecked, hypertension may lead to heart, brain, renal, and other disorders. Have your blood pressure tested often by a health provider so you know your levels. If your blood pressure is high, ask the advice of a health expert. This is crucial in the prevention and treatment of hypertension.

8.Get tested.

Getting yourself tested is a vital step in understanding your health status, particularly when it comes to HIV, hepatitis B, sexually-transmitted infections (STIs) and tuberculosis (TB) (TB). Left untreated, these disorders may lead to severe consequences and even death.

Knowing your status means you will know how to either continue avoiding these illnesses or, if you find out that you're positive, obtain the care and treatment that you need. Go to a public or private health center, wherever you are comfortable, to get yourself tested.

9.Get vaccinated

Vaccination is one of the most efficient strategies to avoid infections. Vaccines interact with your body's natural defences to create protection against illnesses including cervical cancer, cholera, diphtheria, hepatitis B, influenza, measles, mumps, pneumonia, polio, rabies, rubella, tetanus, typhoid, and yellow fever.

In the Philippines, free vaccinations are supplied to children 1 year old and below as part of the Department of Health's regular immunization plan.

Whether you are a teenager or adult, you may ask your physician if to verify your vaccination status or if you wish to get yourself immunized

10. Cover your mouth while coughing or sneezing

Diseases such as influenza, pneumonia and TB are transferred via the air. When an infected individual coughs or sneezes, infectious pathogens may be passed on to others by airborne droplets. When you sense a cough or sneeze coming on, make sure you have covered your mouth with a face mask or use a tissue then discard gently.

If you do not have a tissue nearby when you cough or sneeze, cover your mouth as much as possible with the crook (or the inside) of your elbow.

11. Prevent mosquito bites

Mosquitoes are one of the deadliest creatures in the world. Diseases like dengue, chikungunya, malaria and lymphatic filariasis are spread by mosquitoes and continue to harm Filipinos. You may take basic actions to protect yourself and your loved ones from mosquito-borne infections.

If you're going to a region with known mosquito-borne illnesses, visit a physician for a vaccination to prevent diseases such as Japanese encephalitis and yellow fever or if you need to take antimalarial drugs. Wear light-coloured, long-sleeved shirts and trousers and apply bug repellent. At home, utilize window and door screens, use bed nets and clean your surrounds monthly to remove mosquito breeding places.

12. Follow traffic laws

Road collisions take over one million lives throughout the globe and millions more are wounded. Road traffic injuries are avoidable by a range of measures adopted by the government such as strong laws and enforcement, better infrastructure and vehicle standards, and enhanced post-crash care.

You personally may also avoid road collisions by ensuring that you observe traffic regulations such as using the seatbelt for adults and child restraint for your kids, wearing a helmet while riding a motorbike or bicycle, not drinking and driving, and not using your mobile phone while driving.

13. Drink only clean water

Drinking unclean water may lead to water-borne illnesses such as cholera, diarrhoea, hepatitis A, typhoid and polio. Globally, at least 2 billion people utilize a drinking water source tainted with excrement. Check with your water concessionaire and water refilling station to confirm that the water you're consuming is safe.

 In a location where you are unclear of your water supply, boil your water for at least one minute. This will eliminate hazardous organisms in the water. Let it cool naturally before drinking.

14. Breastfeed infants from 0 to 2 years and beyond

Breastfeeding is the finest technique to offer the optimal diet for babies and infants. WHO advises that moms commence nursing within one hour after delivery. Breastfeeding during the first six months is vital for the infant to grow up healthily.

It is advised that breastfeeding be maintained for up to two years and beyond. Aside from being advantageous to kids, nursing is also excellent for the mother as it decreases the incidence of breast and ovarian cancer, type II diabetes, and postpartum depression.

15 talk to someone that you trust or feeling down or depressed.

is a widespread condition globally with over 260 million individuals afflicted. Depression may show in numerous ways, but it could make you feel hopeless or worthless, or you might think about unpleasant and upsetting ideas a lot or have an overwhelming sensation of suffering. If you're going through this, understand that you are not alone.

Talk to someone you trust such as a family member, friend, coworker or mental health professional about how you feel. If you believe that you are in risk of injuring yourself

16. Take antibiotics only as prescribed

Antibiotic resistance is one of the largest public health problems of our age. When antibiotics lose their potency, bacterial infections become harder to treat, resulting in greater medical expenses, lengthier hospital stays, and increased mortality.

Antibiotics are losing their potency due to abuse and overuse in people and animals. Make sure you only take antibiotics if recommended by a certified health expert. And once prescribed, finish the treatment days as advised. Never share antibiotics.

17. Clean your hands properly

Hand hygiene is crucial not just for health professionals but for everyone.

Clean hands help prevent the transmission of contagious infections. You should handwash using soap and water when your hands are clearly filthy or handrub using an alcohol-based solution.

18. Prepare your meals appropriately

Unsafe food containing hazardous bacteria, viruses, parasites or chemical chemicals, causes more than 200 ailments - ranging from diarrhoea to malignancies. When purchasing food at the market or shop, check the labels or the real product to confirm it is safe to consume. If you are making food, make sure you follow the Five Keys to Safer Food: (1) maintain clean; (2) separate raw and cooked; (3) cook fully; (4) keep food at safe temperatures; and (5) use safe water and raw materials

19. Have frequent check-ups

Regular check-ups may help discover health concerns before they start. Health experts can assist detect and diagnose health concerns early, when your prospects for treatment and cure are greater. Go to your local health center to check out the health services, tests and treatment that are available to you.

(Tips to avoid cancer)

So if you're interested in avoiding cancer, take solace in the idea that modest lifestyle adjustments may make a difference. Consider these cancer-prevention strategies.

<u>1. Don't use tobacco</u>
Using any sort of tobacco puts you on a collision path with cancer. Smoking has been related to several forms of cancer – including cancer of the lung, mouth, throat, larynx, pancreas, bladder, cervix and kidney. Chewing tobacco has been related to cancer of the oral cavity and pancreas. Even if you don't use tobacco, exposure to secondhand smoke could raise your risk of lung cancer.

Avoiding tobacco — or choosing to quit smoking it — is a key aspect of cancer prevention. If you need assistance quitting tobacco, contact your doctor about stop-smoking products and other ways for stopping.

2. Eat a nutritious diet

Although making healthy options at the grocery store and at meals can't ensure cancer prevention, it could lessen your risk. Consider these guidelines:

Eat lots of fruits and veggies. Base your diet on fruits, vegetables and other foods from plant sources — such as whole grains and legumes.

Maintain a healthy weight. Eat lighter and leaner by selecting fewer high-calorie items, including refined carbohydrates and fat from animal sources.

If you prefer to consume alcohol, do so only in moderation The risk of different forms of cancer — including cancer of the breast, colon, lung, kidney and liver — rises with the quantity of alcohol you consume and the length of time you've been drinking frequently.

Limit processed meats. A research by the International Arm for Research on Cancer, the cancer agency of the World Health Organization, indicated that consuming excessive quantities of processed beef may marginally raise the risk of some forms of cancer.

In addition, women who follow a Mediterranean diet enriched with extra-virgin olive oil and mixed nuts could have a lower risk of breast cancer. The Mediterranean diet relies largely on plant-based foods, such as fruits and vegetables, whole grains, legumes, and nuts. People who follow the Mediterranean diet select healthful fats, such as olive oil, over butter and fish instead of red meat.

3. Maintain a healthy weight and remain physically active

Maintaining a healthy weight could lessen the risk of numerous forms of cancer, including cancer of the breast, prostate, lung, colon and kidney.

Physical activity counts, too. In addition to helping you regulate your weight, physical exercise on its own could lessen the risk of breast cancer and colon cancer.

Adults who engage in any level of physical exercise enjoy certain health advantages. But for major health advantages, seek to acquire at least 150 minutes a week of moderate aerobic exercise or 75 minutes a week of strenuous aerobic activity. You may also undertake a mix of moderate and strenuous activities. As a general objective, incorporate at least 30 minutes of physical exercise in your daily routine — and if you can do more, the better.

4. Protect yourself from the sun
Skin cancer is one of the most frequent types of cancer - and one of the most preventable. Try these tips:

Avoid noon sun. Stay out of the sun between 10 a.m. and 4 p.m., when the sun's rays are highest.
Stay in the shade. When you're outside, remain in the shade as much as possible. Sunglasses and a broad-brimmed hat assist, too.

Cover exposed sections. Wear tightly woven, loose fitting clothes that covers as much of your flesh as possible. Opt for vivid or dark hues, which reflect more UV rays than do pastels or bleached cotton.

Don't scrimp on sunscreen. Use a broad-spectrum sunscreen with an SPF of at least 30, especially on overcast days. Apply sunscreen liberally, and reapply every two hours — or more frequently if you're swimming or perspiring.
Avoid tanning beds and sunlamps. These are equally as destructive as natural sunshine.

5. Get vaccine
Cancer prevention involves protection against some viral infections. Talk to

your doctor about immunization against:

Hepatitis B. Hepatitis B may raise the chance of getting liver cancer. The hepatitis B vaccine is recommended for certain adults at high risk — such as adults who are sexually active but not in a mutually monogamous relationship, people with sexually transmitted infections, people who use intravenous drugs, men who have sex with men, and health care or public safety workers who might be exposed to infected blood or body fluids.

Human papillomavirus (HPV) (HPV). HPV is a sexually transmitted virus that may lead to cervical and other genital cancers as well as squamous cell cancers of the head and neck. The

HPV vaccination is recommended for girls and boys aged 11 and 12. The U.S. Food and Drug Administration officially authorized the use of vaccination Gardasil 9 for men and females aged 9 to 45.

6. Avoid dangerous habits

Another effective cancer preventive technique is to avoid dangerous activities that might lead to infections that, in turn, can raise the risk of cancer. For example:

Practice safe sex. Limit your number of sexual partners and wear a condom when you have sex. The more sexual partners you have in your lifetime, the more likely you are to get a sexually transmitted virus — such as HIV or HPV. People who have HIV or AIDS have an increased risk of cancer of the anus, liver and lung. HPV is most typically connected with cervical cancer, but it could also raise the risk of cancer of the anus, penis, throat, vulva and vagina.

Don't share needles. Sharing needles with persons who use intravenous drugs may lead to HIV, as well as hepatitis B and hepatitis C – which can raise the risk of liver cancer. If you're worried about drug usage or addiction, get expert treatment.

<u>7. Get regular medical care</u>
Regular self-exams and tests for several kinds of malignancies — such as cancer of the skin, colon, cervix and breast — might boost your chances of identifying cancer early, when treatment is most likely to be effective.

Ask your doctor about the best cancer screening schedule for you.

Adhering to the above advice and instructions will not only improve your health but also helps you live good and healthy life

www.ingramcontent.com/pod-product-compliance
Lightning Source LLC
Chambersburg PA
CBHW050752180726
48003CB00020B/2346